Frank p Maxwell

THE GLUCOSE ARRANGEMENT:

The Short And Easy Guide To Escape Diabetes

First edition

This book was professionally typeset on Reedsy
Find out more at reedsy.com

Contents

1.

2.

3.

4.

    1.

5.

    1.

6.

    1.

7.

    1.

8.

    1.

Book review

Find balance in your life and in your glucose with the simply following guide on having a better existence

and being a more joyful individual – ideal for anybody hoping to assume command over their body!

With guidance on diet, green living, enhancements, prescription, workout, and customizing the arrangement for ideal outcomes, this book likewise shows peruses how to keep up with long-lasting well-being. Momentous and convenient, The Blood Sugar Solution is the quickest method for getting thinner, forestalling infection, and feeling improved than any time in recent memory.

About the author

Dr.Frank p Maxwell accepts that we as a whole merit an existence of imperativeness – and that we can possibly make it for ourselves. That is the reason he is committed to handling the main drivers of persistent infection by saddling the force of Functional Medicine to change medical care. Dr.Frank p Maxwell and his cooperation consistently engage individuals, associations, and networks to recuperate their bodies and psyches, and work on our social and monetary flexibility.

Dr.Frank p Maxwell is a rehearsing family doctor, an eleven-time New York Times smash hit creator, and a globally perceived pioneer, speaker, teacher, and promoter in his field.

Introduction

Understanding what welcomes corpulence and diabetes is vital.

A double plague of corpulence and type 2 diabetes has struck America. These issues were considerably less normal as of late as quite a while back, so they're not modified into our qualities. Something we're doing or not doing is causing them. What changed to make us inclined to these circumstances? To get it, you really want to think back additional in time - a lot further.

Chapter 1

The Real Causes Of Diabetes

Type 2 Diabetes

Assuming you have Type 2 diabetes, your body's cells can't as expected take up sugar (glucose) from the food sources you eat. Whenever left untreated, Type 2 diabetes can cause such medical issues as coronary illness, kidney sickness, and stroke. You can deal with this infection by making way of life changes, taking meds as well as insulin, and seeing your supplier for customary registrations.

What is Type 2 diabetes?

Type 2 diabetes is a sickness where your body can't utilize energy from food appropriately. Your pancreas produces insulin (a chemical) to assist your cells with utilizing glucose (sugar). Yet, over the long run, your pancreas makes less insulin and the cells oppose the insulin. This causes an excessive amount of sugar to develop in your blood. High glucose levels from Type 2 diabetes can prompt serious medical conditions including coronary illness, stroke, or passing.

Type 1 versus Type 2 diabetes: What's the distinction?

Type 1 diabetes isn't equivalent to Type 2 diabetes. In Type 1 diabetes, your pancreas makes no insulin. In Type 2, your pancreas doesn't make sufficient insulin, and the insulin it is making doesn't necessarily in every case fill in as it ought to. The two sorts are types of diabetes mellitus, meaning they lead to hyperglycemia (high glucose).

Type 2 diabetes typically influences more seasoned grown-ups, however, it's turning out to be more normal in kids. Type 1 diabetes is generally created in kids or youthful grown-ups, yet individuals of all ages can get it.

Who is in danger of creating Type 2 diabetes?

You're bound to foster Type 2 diabetes if you:

- Are you Black, Hispanic, American Indian, Asian American, or Pacific Islander?
- Are more established than 45.
- Have overweight/corpulence.
- Try not to work out.
- Had gestational diabetes while pregnant.
- Have a family background of diabetes.
- Have hypertension.
- Have prediabetes (higher than ordinary glucose, however not sufficiently high to be Type 2 diabetes).

How normal is Type 2 diabetes?

Type 2 diabetes is the most widely recognized type of diabetes. Around 1 of every 10 Americans have the infection. It's the seventh driving reason for death in the U.S.

What are the side effects of Type 2 diabetes?

Side effects of Type 2 diabetes will generally foster gradually over the long haul. They can include:

- Obscured vision.
- Weakness.
- Feeling exceptionally eager or parched.
- Expanded need to pee (as a rule around evening time).
- Slow recuperating of cuts or wounds.
- Shivering or deadness in your grasp or feet.
- Unexplained weight reduction.
- What are the complexities of high glucose levels?
- Possible inconveniences of high glucose levels from Type 2 diabetes can include:
- Stomach-related issues, including gastroparesis.
- Eye issues, including diabetes-related retinopathy.
- Foot issues, including leg and foot ulcers.
- Gum infection and other mouth issues.
- Hearing misfortune.

- Coronary illness.
- Kidney sickness.
- Liver issues, including nonalcoholic greasy liver sickness.
- Fringe neuropathy (nerve harm).
- Sexual brokenness.
- Skin conditions.
- Stroke.
- Urinary lot contaminations and bladder diseases.

Seldom, Type 2 diabetes prompts a condition called diabetes-related ketoacidosis (DKA). DKA is a hazardous condition that makes your blood become acidic. Individuals with Type 1 diabetes are bound to have DKA.

How is Type 2 diabetes analyzed?

The accompanying blood tests assist your medical care supplier with diagnosing diabetes:

Fasting plasma sugary test: checks your blood glucose level. This test is best finished in the workplace in the first part of the day following an eight-hour quick (nothing to eat or drink with the exception of tastes of water).

Arbitrary plasma glucose test: This lab test should be possible at any time without the need to be quick.

Glycosylated hemoglobin testing (A1c) measures your typical glucose levels north of 90 days.

Oral glucose resistance testing checks your glucose levels when you drink a sweet refreshment. The test assesses how your body handles glucose.

How is Type 2 diabetes made due?

There's no remedy for Type 2 diabetes. Be that as it may, you can deal with the condition by keeping a solid way of life and taking prescriptions if necessary. Work with your medical care supplier to deal with your:

Glucose:

A blood glucose meter or nonstop glucose observing (CGM) can assist you with meeting your glucose target. Your medical care supplier may likewise suggest standard A1c tests, oral drugs (pills), insulin treatment, or injectable non-insulin diabetes meds.

Circulatory strain: Lower your pulse by not smoking, practicing routinely, and eating a solid eating regimen. Your medical services supplier might suggest circulatory strain prescriptions like beta-blockers or ACE inhibitors.

Cholesterol: Follow a feast plan low in soaked fats, trans fat, salt, and sugar. Your medical services supplier might suggest statins, which are a sort of medication to bring down cholesterol.

What should a Type 2 diabetes dinner design incorporate?

Ask your medical care supplier or a nutritionist to suggest a dinner plan that is ideal for you. As a general rule, a Type 2 diabetes dinner plan ought to include:

Lean proteins: Proteins low in soaked fats incorporate chicken, eggs, and fish. Plant-based proteins incorporate tofu, nuts, and beans.

Insignificantly handled starches: Refined carbs like white bread, pasta and potatoes can cause your glucose to rapidly increment. Pick carbs that cause a more steady glucose increment, for example, entire grains like oats, earthy colored rice, and entire grain pasta.

No additional salt: Too much sodium, or salt, can build your circulatory strain. Bring down your sodium by keeping away from handled food varieties like those that come in jars or bundles. Pick sans salt flavors and utilize sound oils rather than salad dressing.

Avoid sugars: Avoid sweet food varieties and beverages, like pies, cakes, and pop. Pick water or unsweetened tea to drink.

Non-dull vegetables: These vegetables are lower in carbs, so they don't cause glucose spikes. Models incorporate broccoli, carrots, and cauliflower.

Will I really want a prescription for insulin for Type 2 diabetes?

Certain individuals take prescriptions to oversee diabetes, alongside diet and exercise. Your medical services supplier might suggest oral diabetes meds. These are pills or fluids that you take by mouth. For instance, a medication called metformin helps control how much glucose your liver produces.

You can likewise take insulin to assist your body with utilizing sugar all the more effectively. Insulin comes in the accompanying structures:

Injectable insulin is a shot you give yourself. The vast majority infuse insulin into a beefy piece of their body like their paunch. Injectable insulin is accessible in a vial or an insulin pen.

Breathed insulin is breathed in through your mouth. It is just accessible in a quick-acting structure.

Insulin siphons convey insulin consistently, like how a solid pancreas would. Siphons discharge insulin into your body through a minuscule cannula (meager, adaptable cylinder). Siphons interface with a modernized gadget that allows you to control the portion and recurrence of insulin.

How might I forestall Type 2 diabetes?

You can forestall or postpone Type 2 diabetes by:

Eating a solid eating regimen.

Working out.

Getting more fit.

Customary tests and screenings with your medical care supplier can likewise assist you with holding your glucose under tight restraints.

What is the standpoint for Type 2 diabetes?

Assuming you have Type 2 diabetes, your viewpoint relies on how well you deal with your blood glucose level. Untreated Type 2 diabetes can prompt a scope of hazardous medical issues. Diabetes requires long-lasting administration.

Chapter 2

Five fantasies about diabetes:

There are a ton of legends about diabetes that can truly influence the manner in which individuals ponder the illness. Probably the most predominant diabetes legends defame the condition, which can cause you to feel as if you accomplished something wrong in the event that you have this medical problem. The pressure of dealing with an ongoing conditions (going to constant physical checkups, attempting new prescriptions, managing side effects) can be truly dispiriting, even without the additional load of judgment about your wellbeing.

To assist with standing up against these misperceptions, SELF conversed with specialists about the most widely recognized diabetes fantasies that they hear, alongside the reality behind the legends too.

1. Fantasy: People ought to be humiliated about having diabetes.

You might have a humiliating outlook on having diabetes, however, there are countless purposes behind why having this ailment (or some other) ought not to be dishonorable. First of all, diabetes is inconceivably normal. In excess of 34 million individuals living in the U.S. have the condition, as per the Centers for Disease Control and Prevention. That's around 1 out of 10 individuals. However, regardless of whether it was a less normal condition, the disgrace and shame encompassing diabetes actually wouldn't be legitimate.

There are various explanations behind why diabetes is frequently so slandered, including antifat inclination, bigotry (diabetes is bound to influence minorities more than white individuals), and our social fixation on health, among others. Yet, having diabetes doesn't mean you are some way or another an individual without the condition in any capacity.

In the event that you have type 1 diabetes, your pancreas doesn't make sufficient insulin, a chemical that assists your body with taking sugar from your blood to use as energy. People with type 2 diabetes commonly produce some insulin however can't utilize the chemical really, significance they're insulin-safe, as per the National Institute of Diabetes and Digestive and Kidney Diseases (NIDDK). Type 1 diabetes normally will in general foster significantly sooner than type 2 diabetes.

Specialists don't know what precisely goals the insulin gives that bring about type 1 diabetes, however, they, by and large, accept it happens when your safe framework erroneously goes after solid cells in your body. Type 2 diabetes is the consequence of a blend of hereditary and way of life factors. Having a first-degree relative with diabetes — like your mom or father — expands your gamble of creating the two types of diabetes, as per Jorge Moreno, M.D. an interior medication doctor with Yale Medicine who is likewise board-confirmed in heftiness medication. Either structure can be trashed generally on the grounds that individuals may not figure out diabetes and expect just way of life factors are involved, as indicated by Wendell Malalis, M.D.endocrinologist at Northwestern Medicine Regional Medical Group. "Individuals might feel like [diabetes] was all their issue," he tells SELF.

Since the way of life factors aren't associated with creating type 1 diabetes, it's absolutely impossible to lessen your gamble of fostering the condition. Remaining genuinely dynamic and not being a weight that is restoratively named overweight or fat can diminish an individual's gamble of creating type 2 diabetes by assisting the body with turning out to be more delicate to insulin. Be that as it may, having any genuine command over these sorts of way of life factors is such a great deal not exactly simple or easy. For example, the manner in which you eat and exercise can rely upon where you reside, your timetable, food availability, and how your family raised you to ponder and act around food and wellness. On the off chance that you're a solitary parent who works extended periods of time, for instance, you will most likely be unable to prepare numerous new feasts (which can be more costly and take more time to plan) and exercise frequently. There is no such thing as additionally especially important weight in a vacuum — regardless of how you eat or move your body, factors like your chemicals, rest, and, indeed, hereditary qualities can immensely affect your weight. That is all to say that it's unreasonable and erroneous to fault or pass judgment on anybody for having a condition like diabetes.

All things considered, in the event that you have a family background of type 2 diabetes and need to bring down your sort 2 diabetes hazard (or feel more in charge of your sort 2 diabetes in the event that you have the condition), you might need to converse with your primary care physician about what sensible and feasible way of life changes could significantly impact you.

2. Fantasy: You can foster diabetes on the off chance that you're overweight.

By far most individuals with diabetes have type 2 diabetes. And while weight is one figure creating type 2 diabetes, individuals can have type 2 diabetes at any weight. (There are a lot of individuals in greater bodies who don't have diabetes as well.)

Being overweight is related to insulin obstruction, which can cause type 2 diabetes on the off chance that your glucose remains unreasonably high. Despite the fact that weight file (BMI) is definitely not a decent proportion of individual wellbeing, research shows there's a relationship between having a higher BMI and treating type 2 diabetes. The justification for this isn't completely perceived, yet one explanation could be that certain individuals with a higher BMI have more instinctive fat (or the fat put away in our stomach encompassing our organs). Instinctive fat influences chemical guidelines and having more instinctive fat is related to insulin resistance. But having a higher BMI doesn't ensure you'll get diabetes, and there are individuals with lower BMIs who really do have diabetes.

Past examination shows that certain individuals who were in danger of creating diabetes brought down their possibilities of getting the condition subsequent to shedding pounds through diet and exercise. That is the reason you'll frequently hear that horrible weight is prescribed to assist you with bringing down your possibilities of getting diabetes assuming you're in danger. For certain individuals, weight reduction additionally makes glucose simpler to make due. However, realize that there is no particular measure of weight reduction to bring down the chances of creating diabetes assuming you're in danger or work on your diabetes assuming that you have the condition. Conversing with your doctor can assist you with concluding whether you could profit from shedding pounds and, assuming this is the case, how to do that everything being equal.

3. Legend: You can never eat sugar or carbs assuming that you have diabetes.

On the off chance that you have diabetes Legend: You can never eat sugar or carbs and have gotten an objecting gaze from somebody when you request dessert, then, at that point, you might have encountered the blowback from this fantasy. "There is no great explanation that you need to remove everything," Bithika M. Thompson, M.D.an endocrinologist with the Mayo Clinic in Scottsdale, Arizona, tells SELF. "Everything comes down to adjust."

To keep away from diabetes-related entanglements, you should keep your glucose levels inside an objective range that is intended for you. (Your primary care physician will assist you with setting this objective.) For instance, assuming that you have type 2 diabetes and sugar develops in your blood, then, at that point, you might foster hyperglycemia, or perilously high glucose. Over the long haul high glucose levels can raise your gamble of coronary episode, stroke, and different intricacies.

Despite the fact that you don't have to totally try not to eat carbs or sugar assuming you have diabetes, you might have to roll out a few dietary improvements to keep your glucose levels in your suggested range. For instance, your PCP or dietitian might suggest that you pick complex starches over refined carbs whenever the situation allows, such as deciding on entire wheat bread rather than white bread. Your body separates all starches into glucose (sugar) and uses it for energy. Yet, complex starches take more time to separate, meaning your blood sugars rise all the more leisurely.

You can utilize the glycemic file as an aide for picking food varieties, says Dr. Moreno. The record relegates a number to specific food varieties in view of the fact that they are so prone to make your blood sugars rise.

(The lower the GI number, the more outlandish your glucose will rise.) But remember that the GI is certainly not a thorough rundown and doesn't represent the healthful substance of food sources, similar to whether something has nutrients or fats (which our bodies need). Notwithstanding, one apparatus could assist you with pursuing decisions about what you need to eat.

4. Legend: Insulin is really unsafe.

Insulin assists keep your blood with sugaring low by moving sugar from your circulation system into your phones. Furthermore, keeping a sound glucose is one part of diminishing your possibilities creating other medical issue like coronary illness. In any case, certain individuals erroneously accept that insulin can exacerbate your diabetes.

Insulin is the suggested treatment for the vast majority with type 1 diabetes, as per the American Diabetes Association. People with type 2 diabetes for the most part take different prescriptions as opposed to insulin from the beginning however may have to take insulin in the long haul at last.

The facts really confirm that, similar to any medicine, insulin can accompany incidental effects and expected gambles. Insulin treatment can likewise bring issues like hardship breathing, muscle spasms, and clogging, as per the U.S. Public Library of Medicine.If you unintentionally take a lot of insulin or your primary care physician endorses you a higher portion than what you want, then you might foster low glucose. At the point when this occurs, you could feel exhausted, bad tempered, temperamental, or confounded. For this situation, it's most secure to get clinical help or converse with your primary care physician about how to balance taking an excessive amount of insulin. You might be encouraged to eat and reevaluate your glucose or to get earnest consideration, contingent upon your side effects. By and large, specialists start by giving you low dosages of insulin and step by step expanding your drug to keep away from this incident.

A few examinations show that insulin might be connected to cardiovascular complexities, for example, strokes, in individuals with type 2 diabetes. However, having type 2 diabetes builds your gamble of creating coronary illness, so insulin wasn't really the reason for any heart issues in these examinations. On the off chance that you're stressed over taking insulin, it merits examining your particular worries with your doctor so you can chip away at making a treatment plan you're OK with.

5. Fantasy: You can fix diabetes.

You might have seen notices for items that case to fix diabetes, however truly diabetes is a persistent illness. At the end of the day, there is no diabetes fix.

Yet, you can effectively deal with your condition and even accomplish abatement with the right treatment plan. Certain individuals with type 1 diabetes might bring down their glucose to a nondiabetic range when they're not now consuming any medications after they've proactively been taking drugs for some time. Notwithstanding, this abatement isn't for the most part supportable on the grounds that their body in the long run will not have the option to create insulin all alone, as per the American Diabetes Association.

With type 2 diabetes, you might have the option to accomplish extremely significant stretches of reduction when your glucose levels come to a nondiabetic range without utilizing prescriptions, as indicated by the NIDDK.

In a perfect world, you can have a transparent discussion with your doctor about the most effective way to deal with your glucose, like taking medicine, making dietary changes, or expanding active work. Finding what works for you can take some time, so you might have some experimentation before you notice any glucose changes, as indicated by Dr. Moreno. "Some of the time it takes more than one attempt to get to the underlying driver of the [blood sugar] rise," he says.

Naturally, you might feel separated in the event that you don't know others with diabetes or on the other hand assuming individuals you know trust these legends. While having an ailment can feel actually all-consuming, it tends to be useful to recall that having diabetes isn't a person defect. "It doesn't characterize you," Akankasha Goyal, M.D. clinical associate teacher of medication and endocrinologist at NYU Langone Health, tells SELF.

Chapter 3

Treatment For All kinds Of Diabetes:

Contingent upon what kind of diabetes you have, glucose observation, insulin, and oral medications might be essential for your treatment. Eating a solid eating regimen, remaining at a sound weight And getting customary actual work likewise are significant pieces of overseeing diabetes.

Remedies for a wide range of diabetes

A significant piece of overseeing diabetes — as well as your general wellbeing — is keeping a sound load through a solid eating regimen and exercise plan:

Smart dieting. There's no particular diabetes diet. You'll have to zero in your eating routine on additional natural products, vegetables, lean proteins and entire grains. These are food sources that are high in nourishment and fiber and low in fat and calories. You'll likewise eliminate immersed fats, refined sugars and desserts. It's the best eating plan for the whole family, truth be told. Sweet food varieties are OK sometimes. They should be considered pieces of your feast plan.

Knowing the exact amount to eat can be a test. An enlisted dietitian can assist you with making a feast plan that accommodates your wellbeing objectives, food inclinations and way of life. This will probably incorporate sugar counting, particularly on the off chance that you have type 1 diabetes or use insulin as a feature of your treatment.

Active work. Everybody needs customary oxygen consuming action. This incorporates individuals who have diabetes. Active work brings down your glucose level by moving sugar into your phones, where it's utilized for energy. Active work additionally makes your body more delicate to insulin. That implies your body needs less insulin to move sugar to your cells.

Get your supplier's OK to work out. At a moment in time, pick exercises you appreciate, like strolling, swimming or trekking. What's most significant is making actual work part of your everyday daily practice.

Go for the gold 30 minutes or a greater amount of moderate active work most days of the week, or if nothing else 150 minutes of moderate actual work seven days. Episodes of action can be a couple of moments during the day. On the off chance that you haven't been dynamic for some time, begin gradually and develop gradually. Likewise try not to sit for a really long time. Attempt to get up and move in the event that you've been sitting for over 30 minutes.

Type 1 and Type 2 diabetes Treatment.

Treatment for type 1 diabetes includes insulin infusions or the utilization of an insulin siphon, incessant glucose checks, and carb counting. For certain individuals with type 1 diabetes, pancreas relocation or islet cell relocation might be a choice.

Treatment of type 2 diabetes generally includes a way of life changes, checking of your glucose, alongside oral diabetes medications, insulin, or both.

Checking your glucose

Contingent upon your treatment plan, you might check and record your glucose upwards of four times each day or more regularly assuming that you're taking insulin. A careful routine is the best way to ensure that your glucose level remains within your objective reach. Individuals with type 2 diabetes who aren't taking insulin by and large check their glucose significantly less frequently.

Individuals who get insulin treatment likewise may decide to screen their glucose levels with a consistent glucose screen. Albeit this innovation hasn't yet totally supplanted the glucose meter, it can bring down the number of fingersticks important to check glucose and give significant data about patterns in glucose levels.

Indeed, even with cautious administration, glucose levels can now and again change eccentrically. With assistance from your diabetes treatment group, you'll figure out how your glucose level changes because of food, actual work, drugs, sickness, liquor, and stress. For ladies, you'll figure out how your glucose level changes in light of changes in chemical levels.

Other than day-to-day glucose observing, your supplier will probably prescribe normal A1C testing to quantify your typical glucose level for the beyond 2 to 90 days.

Contrasted and rehashed everyday glucose tests, A1C testing shows better how well your diabetes treatment plan is working generally. A higher A1C level might flag the requirement for an adjustment of your oral medications, insulin routine, or dinner plan.

Your A1C objective might shift relying upon your age and different elements, for example, other ailments you might have or your capacity to feel when your glucose is low. Nonetheless, for the vast majority with diabetes, the American Diabetes Association suggests an A1C of underneath 7%. Ask your supplier what your A1C target is.

Insulin

People with type 1 diabetes require insulin treatment to make due. A lot of people with type 2 diabetes or gestational diabetes additionally need insulin treatment.

Many kinds of insulin are accessible, including short-acting (normal insulin), quick-acting insulin, long-acting insulin, and transitional choices. Contingent upon your requirements, your supplier might endorse a combination of insulin types to use constantly.

Insulin can't be taken orally to bring down glucose since stomach chemicals disrupt insulin's activity. Insulin is in many cases infused utilizing a fine needle and needle or an insulin pen — a gadget that seems to be an enormous ink pen.

An insulin siphon additionally might be a choice. A siphon is a gadget about the size of a little cellphone worn outwardly of your body. A cylinder interfaces the supply of insulin to a cylinder (catheter) that is embedded under the skin of your midsection.

Nonstop glucose screen and insulin siphon

Open spring-up discourse box

A nonstop glucose screen, on the left, is a gadget that acts glucose like clockwork utilizing a sensor embedded under the skin. An insulin siphon joined to the pocket, is a gadget that is worn beyond the body with a cylinder that interfaces the repository of insulin to a catheter embedded under the skin of the mid-region. Insulin siphons are customized to convey explicit measures of insulin constantly and with food.

A tubeless siphon that works remotely is likewise now accessible. You program an insulin siphon to administer explicit measures of insulin. It very well may be acclimated to give out pretty much insulin relying upon dinners, action level, and glucose level.

The Food and Drug Administration has endorsed four counterfeit pancreases for type 1 diabetes.

A fake pancreas is likewise called shut circle insulin conveyance. The embedded gadget interfaces a consistent glucose screen, which checks glucose levels at regular intervals, to an insulin siphon. The gadget naturally conveys the right measure of insulin when the screen demonstrates it's required.

There are more fake pancreas (shut circle) frameworks presently in clinical preliminaries.

Oral or different medications

Once in a while, your supplier might endorse other oral or infused drugs too. Some diabetes drugs assist your pancreas with delivering more insulin. Others forestall the creation and arrival of glucose from your liver, and that implies you want less insulin to move sugar into your cells.

Still, others block the activity of stomach or gastrointestinal chemicals that separate carbs, easing back their assimilation, or making your tissues more delicate to insulin. Metformin (Glumetza, Fortamet, others) is by and large the main medication recommended for type 2 diabetes.

One more class of prescription called SGLT2 inhibitors might be utilized. They work by keeping the kidneys from reabsorbing separated sugar into the blood. All things being equal, the sugar is wiped out in the pee.

Transplantation

In certain individuals who have type 1 diabetes, a pancreas relocation might be a choice. Islet transfers are being concentrated also. With a fruitful pancreas relocation, you would never again require insulin treatment.

However, transfers aren't fruitful 100% of the time. What's more, these methodologies present serious dangers. You want a long period of resistant stifling medications to forestall organ dismissal. These medications can make serious side impacts. Along these lines, transfers are normally saved for individuals whose diabetes can't be controlled or the people who likewise need a kidney relocation.

Bariatric medical procedure

Certain individuals with type 2 diabetes who are corpulent and have a weight list higher than 35 might be helped by having a bariatric medical procedure. Individuals who've had gastric detours have seen significant enhancements in their glucose levels. Yet, this strategy's drawn-out dangers and advantages for type 2 diabetes aren't yet known.

Treatment for gestational diabetes

Controlling your glucose level is crucial for keeping your child solid. It can likewise hold you back from having confusion during conveyance. As well as having a solid eating regimen and practicing routinely, your treatment plan might incorporate checking your glucose. At times, you may likewise utilize insulin or oral medications.

Your supplier will screen your glucose level during work. Assuming your glucose rises, your child might deliver elevated degrees of insulin. This can prompt low glucose just after birth.

Treatment for prediabetes

Assuming you have prediabetes, solid way of life decisions can assist with taking your glucose level back to ordinary. Or on the other hand, it could hold it back from ascending toward the levels found in type 2 diabetes. Keeping a solid load through practice and smart dieting can help. Practicing something like 150 minutes per week and losing around 7% of your body weight might forestall or postpone type 2 diabetes.

Drugs —, for example, metformin, statins, and hypertension prescriptions — might be a possibility for certain individuals with prediabetes and different circumstances like coronary illness.

Difficult situations in a diabetes

Many elements can influence your glucose. Issues may some of the time come up that need care immediately.

High glucose (hyperglycemia)

Your glucose level can ascend for some reasons, including eating excessively, being debilitated, or not taking sufficient glucose-bringing down prescription. Check your glucose level as coordinated by your supplier. What's more, watch for side effects of high glucose, including:

- Peeing frequently
- Feeling thirstier than expected
- Obscured vision
- Sleepiness (weakness)
- Migraine
- Touchiness

Assuming that you have hyperglycemia, you'll have to change your feast plan, drugs, or both.

Expanded ketones in your pee (diabetic ketoacidosis)

On the off chance that your cells are famished for energy, your body might start to separate fat. This spreads the word about harmful acids such as ketones, which can develop in the blood. Watch for the accompanying side effects:

- Queasiness
- Retching
- Stomach (stomach) torment
- A sweet, fruity smell on your breath
- Windedness
- Dry mouth
- Shortcoming

- Disarray
- Trance state

You can check your pee for an overabundance of ketones with a ketones test unit that you can get without a solution. Assuming you have an abundance of ketones in your pee, talk with your supplier immediately or look for crisis care. This frequency is more normal in people with type 1 diabetes.

Hyperglycemic hyperosmolar nonketotic condition

Hyperosmolar condition is brought about by exceptionally high glucose that turns blood thick and sugary.

Side effects of this hazardous condition include:

- A glucose perusing 600 mg/dL (33.3 mmol/L)
- Dry mouth
- Outrageous thirst
- Fever
- Sluggishness
- Disarray
- Vision misfortune
- Mental trips

This condition is found in individuals with type 2 diabetes. It frequently occurs after an ailment. Call your supplier or look for clinical consideration immediately in the event that you have side effects of this condition.

Low glucose (hypoglycemia)

On the off chance that your glucose level dips under your objective reach, it's known as low glucose (hypoglycemia). Assuming you're ingesting medications that bring down your glucose, including insulin, your glucose level can drop for some reasons. These incorporate skirting a feast and getting more active work than ordinary. Low glucose likewise happens if you take a lot of insulin or an over-the-top glucose-bringing-down prescription that makes the pancreas hold insulin.

Check your glucose level routinely and watch for side effects of low glucose, including:

- Perspiring
- Instability
- Shortcoming
- Hunger
- Wooziness
- Cerebral pain
- Obscured vision
- Heart palpitations
- Touchiness
- Slurred discourse
- Tiredness
- Disarray
- Swooning
- Seizures

Low glucose is best treated with carbs that your body can retain rapidly, like natural product juice or glucose tablets.

Chapter 4

Diabetes Cordial Food Choices

Diabetes cordial food choices are just about as close as your kitchen.

At the point when you have prediabetes or diabetes, a sound diabetes dinner plan is critical to dealing with your glucose. Here and there it very well may be precarious to know which food sources and beverages are great decisions, however, these 10 picks can assist with holding your numbers under wraps.

1. Beans (Of Any Kind!)

Whether they're lentils, kidneys, pinto, dark, or garbanzo, beans are a low-glycemic record food. That implies their carbs are slowly delivered so they're less inclined to cause glucose spikes. They're gainful to such an extent that one investigation discovered that eating a day-to-day cup of beans for a considerable length of time as a component of a low-glycemic file diet brought down HbA1c by a portion of a rating point.

Attempt it! Trade in beans for around 50% of the meat in tacos or your number one stew recipe.

2. Apples

You could feel that there's no room in a diabetic feast plan for a natural product, however, apples are likewise low glycemic. Holding back nothing apples that are low or medium on the glycemic file is one method for overseeing glucose levels. Furthermore, eating an apple daily has its advantages - they are high in fiber, L-ascorbic acid as well as sans fat! Also a versatile and simple nibble choice.

Attempt it! Throw an apple in your lunch sack or get one between feasts. Prepare them and add cinnamon for a warm treat.

3. Almonds

These crunchy nuts are plentiful in magnesium, a mineral that might be useful to your body to utilize its own insulin all the more successfully. Take a stab at working more almonds into your eating regimen — one ounce (around 23 entire nuts) supplies almost 20% of your day-to-day portion of this glucose-adjusting mineral. Besides, nuts like almonds are high in monounsaturated unsaturated fats, protein, and fiber, which makes them an extraordinary method for overseeing blood glucose levels.

Attempt it! For sound eating in a hurry, pack one-ounce bits of almonds into single-serve compartments.

4. Spinach

This significant vegetable has only 21 calories for every cooked cup and is loaded up with glucose cordial magnesium and fiber. Furthermore, you can appreciate spinach crude, sautéed with olive oil, cooked, or even mixed. Pursuing it is a flexible decision as well!

Attempt it! Prepare a stacking modest bunch of child spinach into your next smoothie or use it instead of lettuce in a plate of mixed greens.

5. Chia Seeds

You could have heard that losing or overseeing weight is quite possibly everything you can manage to further develop your glucose. Chia seeds can assist with that. In one review, individuals with diabetes who added about an ounce of chia seeds per 1,000 calories per day to a calorie-controlled diet for quite some time shed four pounds and managed an inch-and-a-half from their waistlines. Besides being loaded with fiber, these pearls additionally contain protein and give 18% of your suggested day-to-day admission of calcium.

Attempt it! Join a quarter-cup of chia seeds with one cup of one-percent or nonfat milk and one-half cup of diced natural product. Refrigerate for the time being and appreciate breakfast the following morning.

6. Glucerna Shakes and Bars

While you're having a furious day eating right can be troublesome. Glucerna shakes and bars can make things simpler. Made by Abbott, they have mixes of starches that are gradually processed and consumed to assist with limiting glucose spikes. With less than 200 calories for each shake and under 160 calories for every bar, they're a shrewd, segment-controlled decision.

Attempt it! Stash a couple of Glucerna bars or shakes in your vehicle or work area cabinet so you'll continuously have a solid bite close by — regardless of how occupied your day is.

7. Blueberries

Another natural product choice: the proof of the medical advantages of eating blueberries is really convincing. Blueberries contain intensifiers that have been displayed to assist with lessening the gamble of coronary illness and assist with further developing how your body utilizes insulin. One review showed that eating what might be compared to around two cups of blueberries every day superior insulin responsiveness in overweight individuals with insulin opposition. They're likewise an extraordinary wellspring of fiber and different supplements like L-ascorbic acid and cell reinforcements, and blueberries are a phenomenal method for getting your fill.

Attempt it! Take a half-cup of new blueberries (or thawed-out, frozen blueberries) and spoon over plain, unsweetened yogurt. Or on the other hand, add a cup of blueberries to your smoothie.

8. Cereal

Cereal isn't only really great for your heart. It can help your glucose as well. Steel cut and moved oats have a low-glycemic file and are a preferred decision over food sources, for example, white bread, grain chips, or corn drops. Simply remember that while steel cut and moved oats are extraordinary picks, profoundly handled moment and fast oats will more often than not be higher on the glycemic record so they're not as glucose amicable.

Attempt it! Select steel or moved oats cooked oats with blueberries for a generous, hot breakfast.

9. Turmeric

This brilliant flavor contains curcumin, a substance that might keep your pancreas solid and forestall prediabetes from transforming into Type 2 diabetes. How well does it function? At the point when scientists gave members, who had prediabetes 1500 mg of a curcumin supplement day to day or a fake treatment for quite some time, 16% of individuals in the fake treatment bunch proceeded to become diabetic, while the whole curcumin bunch remained diabetes free. This study gives some understanding into how an old zest like turmeric can assist with further developing how the body can work on its aversion to insulin.

Attempt it! Curry powder is loaded up with turmeric. Sprinkle some into your next veggie pan sear for a curcumin kick or converse with medical services proficient about utilizing an enhancement.

10. Chamomile Tea

Chamomile tea has for quite some time been utilized for different sicknesses. Existing examination shows that it has cell reinforcement and anticancer properties, and a new report has found that it might assist you with dealing with your glucose levels too. At the point when members in the review drank one cup of chamomile tea after dinner three times each day for quite some time, they showed a decrease in glucose levels, insulin, and insulin opposition.

Chapter 5

Turning Around The Diabetes Pandemic:

1. Get the right tests. Most specialists center around fasting glucose. This is really an unfortunate mark of diabetes. The best test to coax out the condition is an insulin reaction test where insulin levels are estimated fasting and afterward 1 and 2 hours after a glucose drink. Request this test from your PCP.

2. Become brilliant about nourishment

In spite of the media publicity and the appearing disarray among specialists, the essentials of sustenance are very basic. Kill sugar and handle carbs, incorporate entire genuine food varieties like lean protein (chicken or fish), veggies, nuts, seeds, beans and entire grains.

3. Get the right enhancements. There has as of late been a furor of negative reports about supplements. The greater part of them are unwarranted. Supplements are a fundamental piece of treating diabetes. A decent multivitamin, vitamin D, fish oil, and unique glucose adjusting supplements like alpha lipoic corrosive, chromium polynicotinate, biotin, cinnamon, green tea catechins, and PGX (a super fiber) ought to likewise be incorporated.

4. Get loose. Stress is a significant unnoticed supporter of insulin obstruction and glucose irregularity. Press your respite button consistently with profound breathing, perception, yoga, and other unwinding strategies.

5. Get rolling. Beside changing your eating regimen, practice is presumably the absolute best drug for diabetes. Stroll for somewhere around 30 minutes consistently. For some purposes, 30-an hour of more energetic vigorous activity 4-6 times each week might be essential.

6. Get spotless and green. Ecological poisons likewise add to diabetes. Channel your water, search for green cleaning items, and stay away from plastics when you can.

7. Get individual. While the means above will resolve 80% of the issues with diabetes, some might have to find extra ways to enhance key regions of their science. Keep in mind, the medication representing things to come is private medication. Search out your own organic irregular characteristics and search for ways of tending to them.

8. Get associated. Research is starting to show that we get better more successfully when we get together. Welcome your companions, families, and neighbors to change their weight control plans and way of life alongside you. Together we can all reclaim our well-being.

Conclusion

It's critical to screen diabetes intently on the off chance that you're debilitated. Indeed, even a typical virus can be perilous on the off chance that it impedes your insulin and glucose levels. Make a "day off" plan with your medical services supplier so you know how frequently to check your glucose and what prescriptions to take.

Contact your supplier immediately on the off chance that you experience:

- Disarray or cognitive decline.
- Fever of 100°F or higher.
- High glucose for over 24 hours.
- Sickness and spewing for over four hours.
- Issues with equilibrium or coordination.
- Serious agony anyplace in your body.
- Inconvenience moving your arms or legs.

Type 2 diabetes is an illness where your body doesn't make sufficient insulin and can't utilize sugar in the manner in which it ought to. Sugar, or glucose, develops in your blood. High glucose can prompt serious unexpected problems. However, Type 2 diabetes is reasonable. Normal activity and a sound eating routine can assist you with dealing with your glucose. You may likewise require a drug or insulin. On the off chance that you have Type 2 diabetes, you ought to screen your glucose at home routinely and remain nearby with your medical care supplier.